Secrets Of Good Health

Olatundun Solomon

olatundunsolomon@gmail.com

Olatundun Solomon has distinction in the program Diploma in Nursing and Patient Care.

He has distinction in the program Diploma in Human Nutrition.

He has Honor code certificate from Karolinska Institutet in edx. The course is KIBEHMEDx:

Behavioral Medicine: A Key to

Better Health.

From the University of

Queensland in edx he has the

certificate BIOIMG101x:

Introduction to Biomedical

Imaging.

From Harvard University in edx

he has the certificate HSPH-

HMS214x: Fundamentals of

Clinical Trials.

From Harvard University he also

has the certificate PH201x:

Health and Society. From the

University of Texas System in

edx he has the certificate 4.01x:

Take Your Medicine - The

Impact of Drug Development.

Secrets Of Good Health:

There are many principles to be taking concerning health in order to have good health. The human body has eyes, tongue, teeth, throat, hands, legs, intestines, lungs, heart, kidney, nose, ear, skin and many other parts of the body. There are many secrets to know that should be done medically for the body to have good health.

The human body require things

that are normal. When it is over

normal it is not good for the

body or when it is below normal

it is not good for the body. For

example, clean water is good

for the body. It is good to drink

clean water. But when this

clean water is over taken in, it is

not good for the body. It can

make someone to be

uncomfortable. Even good food

when it is over eaten above

normal it can cause vomiting to

occur and it can make

somebody not to be

comfortable. It usually cause

negative effects to the body. It

can cause obesity, diabetes

mellitus and heart diseases. This

can result due to over storage of

glucose in the body. When

glucose is very much in the body,

it can make glucose to be much

in the urine(diabetes). When glucose is very much in the body it is then start to be converted into fat which can cause obesity and heart problem. This is due to malnourishment.

When good food is eaten below normal, that is very little. This result to malnutrition. This is because the nutrients are very little because the food is very little. This can cause kwashiorkor, under weight,

fatigue, electrolyte imbalance

and anemia(blood level below

normal).

These are secrets that should be

known and take action on them

for the body to have good

health:

1. Secrets about sweet food:

Sweet food such as sugar, sweet

potato and other sweet food is

that, they give energy to the body. This is because of the presence of glucose. Glucose is monosaccharide. From the word saccharide means sweet. When this food is eaten moderately it is very good for the body to have good health. But when this food is over consumed and leaving other food not eaten like lemon,

lime,

fish,

beans,

vegetable oil,

iodized salt. Iodized salt is

needed very little in food.

When it is over consumed

in high quantity, it makes

the heart to beat very fast.

This is because of sodium

ion and chlorine ion that is

present. When the heart

beats very fast, it is

hypertension.

Hypertension can cause death. It is therefore, expected to put a little amount of salt in the food for hypertension to be prevented. The iodine in the iodized salt helps to prevent goitre. This is because the thyroid gland will not swell to form goitre because of the

presence of iodine.

In continuation of sweet

food. When it is over

consumed, the glucose will

store up in the liver and

also in the muscles. This

continue storing of glucose

will make the glucose to

be converted into adipose

tissues (fatty tissues). This

will eventually make the

body to be very big in size.

This is obesity. The fat that

is formed can start to form

at the inner wall of the

artery. This is

atherosclerosis. This will

make the blood pressure

to rise and form

hypertension. This is

because, the narrower the

vessel the higher the blood

pressure. Because the

blood vessels are
narrowed, hypertension
will then occur. It is
therefore good to eat
sweet food moderately
and have exercise for
obesity not to occur.
Exercise is good because,
the body will have
increase in temperature.
This increase in
temperature will lead to

the burning down of fat.
This will then prevent and
treat obesity. After eating
sweet food, it is good to
brush the teeth because
the remnants in the mouth
can be converted into acid
that can cause the teeth to
demineralize and increase
the acidic level of the body.

2. Secrete of spices: Spices are antiseptics and antibiotics. The secrets about this is that, the microorganisms for example bacteria. Because of the spicy effect of the spices such as ginger, curry and other spices makes them to be uncomfortable and the spicy effect on them makes them to not live in the body to cause disease to the body. But the

spicy effect should be felt

enough in the food when there

is bacterial infection. But when

there is bacteria infection and

the spices is used in a very little

amount the effect of the spice

will not be felt much in the food.

This will make it not to be very

effective because the

concentration is little. After

using the spice in a quantity

that is felt during an infection

period, after the infection is over, it is expected to use spices in food moderately in order for the spice not to have adverse effects to the body.

3. Secrets about bathing:

Bathing is very good to the body. This will make any disease causing microorganism to be washed away from the skin.

Bacteria, viruses and fungi are washed away by using soap and water during bathing. Bacteria acts for decay to occur. It can act on the skin by feeding on it and this can cause disease. When bath is taken, the bacteria is washed away and skin disease is prevented. When there is no disease causing microorganisms on the skin it is good to take bath. This will prevent a place that is suitable

for bacteria to act. Bacteria is

very effective in dirty

environment, this is because

bacteria act for decay to occur

and this is pathogenic to the

body. It is good to bath in the

morning and in the night before

sleeping. This will prevent dirty

environment for bacteria to act

on. Bathing in the morning and

night is good because when the

body sweat, bacteria act on the sweat. This makes the sweat to smell. When the sweat is not washed away it result to body odour and skin infection. After wearing clothes, some parts of the body is exposed such as the hands, head and neck. These places can have contact with aerobic bacteria. When bath is taken pathogens are washed away, skin infection is

prevented and body odour is
prevented.

4. Secrets of sour fruits:

Sour fruits such as lime and
lemon are very good for the
body. It is very good as
antibiotics. This is because, sour
fruit is acidic. Because of the
acidic nature, it helps to treat
disease caused by pathogens.

When it is eaten more during an infection, it makes the body to be affected by such and the pathogens will not be able to thrive. This will make treatment to occur. But after treatment has occurred, it is expected to eat lemon or lime moderately in order for the body not to have disease that is due to acidic condition. For example, acidosis. When there is no pathogens that infect the body and acidic

fruits are over eaten, it can

cause the teeth to demineralize,

that is calcium in the teeth will

start to reduce. This will make

the teeth to be weak and

unhealthy. Because the teeth is

not strong it can easily break.

When the acidic level of the

body is very high it can cause

ulcer. This is because acid can

burn. This can cause the inner

layer of the stomach to burn

and cause injury, this is stomach

ulcer. It can cause the inner

layer of the esophagus to burn

and there is injury. This is

esophageal ulcer. And when the

intestine is affected, it is called

intestinal ulcer.

5. Secrets about water:

Water is very important to the

body. The human body

dehydrate when there is loss of

water from the body through

feces, sweating and urination. It

occurred because water is

present in feces, sweat and

urine. It is expected to drink

enough water to replace the

water that as passed out from

the body. After drinking enough

water, it will make the body to

hydrate. Drinking of clean water

is important, because dirty

water cause infection to occur

to the body. Cholera occur and

also diarrhea due to dirty water

consumption. This is because of

the bacteria that is present. The

bacteria will feed on the

nutrients of the body and starve

the body of nutrients. The

bacteria will multiply in the

body. This will make the body

to be sick. It is therefore

expected for somebody to drink

clean water. Drinking of clean

water helps in the digestion of

food. It helps in preventing

constipation (inability to

deficate). Drinking of clean

water also enable the flow of

blood to be normal. This is

because dehydration is

prevented and the blood will

not be too thick. Drinking of

clean water also helps in

bringing the temperature of the

body to a normal, after

exposure to a very high

temperature area. This is

because water has the ability to

reduce high temperature.

6. Secrets concerning the sun:

The sun is very important. Early

morning sun gives vitamin D to

the body. Vitamin D helps the

bone to absorb calcium. This

makes the bone to be

mineralized. This increase the

density of the bone. This makes

the bone to be strong and

healthy. But it is good not to

stay under the hot sun. From

the sun is UV1 and UV2, both

are ultraviolet rays.

These rays can cause mutation

of the DNA in the skin. It is good

to not stay under the hot sun as

hobby. When the skin is

exposed to the hot sun, it can

lead to changes in the DNA of

the skin. This is mutation, which result to cancer of the skin. This should not be misunderstood with the early morning sun that gives vitamin D to the body that is very beneficial. The mutation occur from the hot sun because Ultraviolet rays (UV1 and UV2) has the ability to mutate the DNA, just like how X-ray has the ability to mutate. The sun can also cause dehydration to occur. It is very important to

wear cloths, cap, shoes and also

to open the umbrella, this helps

to prevent skin cancer and body

dehydration. When the body is

exposed to the hot sun,

dehydration occur due to the

high temperature from the sun.

This high temperature makes

water to evaporate from the

body. This cause dehydration to

occur to the body. It is needful

to drink enough water, for

hydration to occur.

7. Secrets of teeth brushing:

Teeth brushing is very good to

make the teeth clean and

healthy. When the teeth is not

washed with fluoridated

toothpaste and toothbrush. It

makes the teeth dirty. This

allow bacteria to decompose

remnants of food in the mouth.

This will cause teeth

discoloration. This will make

tooth caries to occur. When

teeth is not brushed when

sugary food is eaten, the

bacteria in the mouth convert it

into acid and this acid

demineralize the teeth. This can

make the teeth to have cavity.

After cavitation of the teeth it

result to pain that is not

comfortable. It is good to brush
the teeth with fluoridated
toothpaste and toothbrush. And
clean the mouth with clean
water. This will not make food
remnants to be present in the
mouth, that can be converted
into acid. That can demineralize
the teeth and cause cavity.
When the mouth is not brushed
regularly in the morning after
meal and at night after last

meal, the caries that form on

the teeth is the food remnants

that as been decomposed by

bacteria and it coat on the teeth.

When the teeth is properly

washed, this is prevented. This

will not make tooth ache to

occur that is caused by low level

of blood to the teeth after tooth

cavitation as occurred. Pain

usually occur to the part of the

body that is having below

normal blood supply. In tooth
cavitation, the hole in the tooth
cause less blood supply to the
teeth and this cause pain. When
the teeth is properly taken good
care of this will not occur. When
the teeth is clean mouth odour
is prevented. What causes
mouth odour is when the teeth
is not brushed with fluoridated
toothpaste and clean water. The
remnants of food in the mouth

will be decomposed by bacteria

and this will cause bad breath.

When somebody speaks it will

then bring discomfort to the

person that is having mouth

odour and also to the person

that he or she is speaking to. It

is therefore good to prevent this

by brushing the teeth after

breakfast and brushing the

teeth after meal at night. This

will not allow remnant of food

to be in the mouth that can cause mouth odour after it has been decomposed by bacteria. Remnants of food will not be present in the mouth. Therefore, mouth odour is prevented.

8. Secrets about sleep: The body has circadian rhythm. This is twenty four hours. When there is no proper sleep the rhythm is

affected. This is not healthy to the body. When there is lack of sleep at night it cause black eye to occur. When there is black eye the white part of the high that is called the sclera will become reddish. The reddishness indicate symptom of lack of sleep. When there is lack of sleep the body is not refreshed using the circadian rhythm. This will make the body to be weak and the brain is also affected, it will not be sharp as normal because of the circadian rhythm.

9. Secrets about infection: Infection is caused by bacteria, viruses, fungi and other disease causing microorganisms. This occur when pathogens (disease causing microorganisms) stays on the skin, stays in the mouth after putting dirty objects into

the mouth, stays in the stomach and the intestines after swallowing dirty food and not well cooked food that contain pathogens and also disease causing microorganisms can stay on wounds that are exposed to the air. This is because some bacteria can stay in the air(aerobic bacteria). When food is not covered properly, it can cause pathogens to be found on it.

What the pathogens does is that they feed on the host(the person that is infected). The pathogens that are found on the wound that is exposed, feed on the wound. This will make the wound not to heal easily and it will make the wound to smell. This will make the wound to keep on expanding because, the pathogens are feeding on it. When food has disease causing microorganisms in it, and the food is eaten. This will make the pathogens infect the stomach and intestine. The blood also will be infected (hemosepsis). This will make the pathogens to feed on the blood and this will make the blood level to be below normal(anemia). For example, plasmodium parasite feed on the blood. This will make high temperature to occur (fever). Because oxygen is transported to different parts of the body, by the help of hemoglobin which is present in the blood. The malaria parasite plasmodium feed on the hemoglobin. This makes the body to not have enough hemoglobin to transport oxygen. The more the parasite continue to feed on the hemoglobin, the more the fever continue to be severe. It is good to go to the hospital early so that the doctor can prescribe antimalarial drug. And it is expected for the patient to follow the prescription.

To prevent infection of disease causing microorganisms, it is expected to have body hygiene. This makes the body to be clean and pathogens are washed away. It is also good to cook food such as beef, chicken, turkey, goat meat, ram meat and fish very well. This makes any pathogen that is present to not be alive in the food. This will make the food to not have negative effect to the body. It is good to drink clean water. This makes pathogens to not be present in it. This makes the body to be free from pathogens.

It is also expected in the hospital to use different syringes for patients during therapy (treatment). This will not allow disease to be transferred from person to person.

10. Secrets about drug:

Drug prescription is done by doctors in the hospital. There is dosage that is expected to be taken by the patients. It is expected for the patient to take the correct dosage so that harmful effect will be prevented. Synthetic drugs are made from chemicals. When the drug is taken above the correct prescribed dosage, it cause harmful effect which is toxic to the body. And when the drug is taken below the correct prescribed dosage it makes the drug ineffective. The drug act on receptors in the body that makes the drug to have it's efficacy in the body. It is good to take the correct dosage so that the receptors can be activated well, in order for therapy (treatment) to occur.

11. Secrets of carbohydrates:
Carbohydrate food are rice, wheat, yam, potato and maize. Carbohydrate food gives energy to the body. Carbohydrate is broken down to glucose and stored in the muscles and liver. Glycogen is the form in which glucose is stored in the liver. When carbohydrate is eaten above normal, that is in excess. This makes the extra glucose to

be converted into fat and stored in the body. This makes the body to be obese. When carbohydrate is eaten moderately and other food is not eaten, this result to kwashiorkor. The head will be big(cephalomegally). And the belly will be big.

12. Secrets of vegetable oil:

Vegetable oil is very good for

the body. It contains

unsaturated fatty acid.

Vegetable oil does not mix or

dissolve in water. It has smooth

lubricating ability that makes

the joints to move freely and

friction is prevented. This makes

wear and tear not to occur to

the joints. This prevent arthritis.

Avocado fruit and soybeans has

unsaturated fatty acid. Avocado oil and soy oil lubricate the joints and arthritis is prevented. But it is expected for the food (avocado and soybeans) be eaten moderately for the oil be enough for arthritis to be prevented.

13. Secrets of vegetables:

Vegetable is good for the good

health of the body. Green leafy

vegetable has folic acid. This

folic acid is good for blood

production from the bone

marrow. This prevent

anemia(blood level below

normal). Green leafy vegetables

also prevent cancer of the

colon(large intestine). This is

because it has a lot of fiber that

act like sponge. This helps in

cleaning up the walls of the

colon. This prevent cancerous cell formation. Green vegetables also helps when the acidic level of the body is high that can cause body pain is brought down.

14. Secrets about protein: Protein is food that is for growth and development. Protein contains amino acid

residue that helps to build up the body. This makes the structure of the body to be well developed. Growth hormone also assist in the growth of the body. It is good for children to eat a lot of protein, such as beef, egg, chicken, fish, turkey and beans. This makes the children to not have defect in growth. Auxopathy(disease that relate to growth) is prevented. For growth to occur to the muscles,

myocytes are produced. For

growth to occur to the bones,

osteoblast and osteocytes are

produced. For growth to occur

to the nerves, neurons are

produced and for growth to

occur to the cartilage,

chondrocytes are produced.

Protein helps in the general

growth of the body.

15. Secrets about fruits: Fruits has a lot of vitamin that are very important to the body. The vitamins are water soluble vitamins and fat soluble vitamins. Water soluble vitamins can dissolve in water and fat soluble vitamins can be absorbed in fat in the intestine. Too much consumption of fat soluble vitamins store up in the fatty tissues of the body. And

this is harmful to the body by causing vitaminosis. When fat soluble vitamins are gotten by eating balance diet moderately, it result to avitaminosis(vitaminosis is not present). Fat soluble vitamins are vitamin A, D, E and K. Water soluble vitamins are vitamin B and C. The body needs this vitamins in other for the body to function normally. When the body functions normally, the immune

level of the body will be high.

This will make the body to be

able to fight against diseases.

This is why vitamins helps the

body to be able to fight against

diseases. The white blood

cells(leukocytes) fight against

diseases. Too little consumption

of fruits and balance diet will

make the body to not have

enough vitamins. Eaten of

balance diet is good. It is also

good to eat it not to little or

over eating. Over eaten will

make the body not to be

comfortable. It is good to eat

balance diet moderately. Apart

from vitamins that fruits gives

to that body, fruits also has a lot

of fiber. When you cut the fruit,

you will be able to see the fibers.

This fibers makes the food not

to be very fast absorbed into

the body. This makes obesity to

be prevented and the body

weight is regulated normally.

The fibers also helps to clean up

the large intestine because it act

like sponge. This makes cancer

of the large intestine to be

prevented. Some fruits are very

bitter. Because of the bitter

effect, microorganisms find it

uncomfortable. This makes

pathogens to not feed on the

blood. When they do not feed

on the blood, they will not be

able to live in the blood. This

will then treat diseases that are

caused by pathogens. This is

why bitter fruits are good for

the treatment of fever. For

example for the treatment of

typhoid fever, malaria fever and

other types of fever. Bitter

fruits are also good to be taken

during pathogen infections.

Bitter fruits also helps to

prevent infections by pathogens.

16. Secrets of cloth washing:

When clothes are used and are

not washed, it will cause

bacteria and other

microorganisms to be on it.

When the clothes are worn

outside, there can be bacteria in

the air(aerobic bacteria) that

can be on the clothes. The

clothes can touch places that

pathogens are present. The

clothes can have contact will

pathogens that cause

communicable diseases.

Because of this reasons, it is

very crucial to wash to clothes

with soap and water. This will

make the pathogens to be

washed away. It is also good to

dry clothes under the sun and

make sure that the clothes are

well dry before wearing.

Disease causing microorganisms do not like to act in a very dry environment. They love to act in a moist environment.

17. Secrets about exercise:

Exercise is very important to the body. This helps to regulate the body structure. When different parts of the body is used well, those parts develops well.

When some body parts are not

used well it makes those parts

not to develop well. When a

part of the body is well used ,

the body will develop in order

to meet that situation for the

body to adapt to that condition.

For example, when you are

jogging. The body will produce

more calcium, phosphorus,

magnesium and also collagen

that will increase the density of

the bone. This will help to

prevent osteoporosis and

osteopenia. This will therefore

make the bone to be strong and

healthy.

When there is lack of exercise it

result to atrophy of the body

parts. This is, the body parts will

reduce. This is because the body

will not be able to develop that

part that is disused. The body

will want to adapt to that

disused part of the body and

this will make that part not to

develop.

18. Secrets about cancer:

There are two types of cancer.

They are benign cancer and

malignant cancer. Benign cancer

does not spread to other parts

of the body while malignant

cancer does. The cause of

cancer is due to the normal

basic inheritance information

the DNA is changed. The

changed DNA will multiply. This

will then make the normal DNA

be replaced by the mutated.

This can cause death. It is very

important to prevent

carcinogens(agents that can

cause cancer) from affecting the

body. Carcinogens are

preservatives in food, colorants in food, UV1 and UV2 from the hot sun, smokes and other additives in food.

19. Secrets about animal fat:

Animal fat when eaten as food, this makes fat to be stored in the body. This makes over weight to occur. This also makes fat to be found on the walls of the arteries. Arteries are vessels that helps in the movement of blood. When this fat are found in the walls of the arteries, this makes the walls to be narrow. The narrower the vessels becomes the higher the blood pressure. This then result to hypertension. If the animal fat is eaten continually as food it can cause stroke and death. It can cause stroke because the blood supply to the brain will be

reduced. This will make the

oxygen to the brain to be

reduced. This is because oxygen

is in the blood and the blood

that is reaching the brain is very

little. When the brain is not well

nourished the brain will not

function properly. This will then

make the brain not to be able to

sense the legs effectively and it

will result to stroke. This is

ischaemic stroke, because the

the inner lumen(tunica intima)

is covered by fat. And there is

insufficient supply of blood to

the brain. This leads to

insufficient supply of oxygen to

the brain. Note very clearly that

oxygen makes the brain to be

alive. Lack of oxygen to the

brain, result to brain death.

20. Secrets about kidney stone(renolith) and gall stone(cholecystolith): Kidney stone and gall stone occur as a result of undissolved drug in the body. It can also occur due to reaction of chemicals in the body. When there is too high the level of calcium and phosphorus in the body it can be formed. Calculi(Stone) can also form in different parts of the body, such as in the salivary gland, urethra and ureter. To prevent calculi formation in the body, it is expected to drink enough water. This helps to make any chemical that will want to cause calculi to be urinated. When there is calculi in the ureter, this will make urine passage to be very little. Because of the difficulty to pass urine this will make pain to develop. When there is calculi in the kidney, this will make ultrafiltration of blood by the kidney to be difficult. This can then result to the loss of important ions that should have been absorbed into the blood to be urinated. This can eventually lead to the use of dialysis machine. It is therefore very important to drink sufficient water for calculi to be

prevented from forming in the
body.

21. Secrets about honey: Honey
is sweet to the taste, this makes
it good to be used as appetizer.
Also sugar is used as appetizer.
Brown sugar is very good to be
used, because it has not yet
been refined. The refined sugar
has less nutrient compared to

the brown sugar. Honey is good

also because it is fructose, it can

be easily digested by the body

and is good for the health.

Sugar can easily raise the blood

glucose level and cause diabetes

mellitus. Diabetes mellitus

means passage of sweet urine.

Therefore too much sugar in the

diet is not good. Too little sugar

in the diet is not good, it can

make the body to be weak. This

is because sugar is carbohydrate

that gives energy to the body.

Symptoms of diabetes mellitus

is frequent passage of urine and

there can be seen ants in the

place that the urine is. This is

because the urine is sweet.

There is loss of gucose in the

urine. There is loss of weight.

There is the smell of acetone.

When there is frequent

urination, this makes loss of

water to occur and the body will

dehydrate. It is therefore good

to eat healthy diet and to do

exercise. Healthy diet makes

eating of more of sugar and

carbohydrates not to occur.

Eating of more of sugar and and

carbohydrates can cause

diabetes mellitus. It is good to

eat balance diet. Eating of fish,

fruits, vegetables, beans, milk,

egg, wheat, rice, potato, yam

and maize is good. These should

be eaten moderately.

22. Secrets about house

cleaning: It is good to keep the

house clean. This prevent

pathogens to be present.

Pathogens usually stays in dirty

place. For example, in dirty

toilet, on dirty chairs, in dirty

mattress, on dirty wall, in dirty

rug, on dirty table and on dirty

carpet. When the house is well

cleaned, it prevent disease

causing microorganisms. When

the house is not clean, when

ever the dirt's are touched it

makes infection to occur to the

body. When the house is not

clean and it is dirty, it can result

to psychopathy. This is because

the mind set of the person

having the house will not be

comfortable in the house when

he look at the dirts. It is

therefore, good to make sure

that the house is clean.

23. Secrets of preventing

diseases from unwashed fruit:

Unwashed fruit is not good to

be eaten. This is because, from

where the fruit is brought, it has

been exposed. There are

aerobic bacteria in the air that

might have come in contact

with it. The fruit might have

come in contact with dirty

substances that can make

pathogens to be on the fruit.

When the fruit is eaten without

washing it, it makes the mouth,

stomach, intestine and various

parts of the body to be infected.

This can lead to coughing and

other diseases to occur. It is

therefore important to wash

the fruit thoroughly with clean

water for any pathogen that is

present on it be washed away.

This will make the fruit edible.

And diseases will be prevented

from occurring to the body.

24. Secrets of preventing hair

from falling: Hair falling may be

normal or not. When it is

normal, is during bald head. But

when it is not normal the hair

will keep on falling. This can be
as a result of hair infection. It
can also result from skin
infection. It is good to wash the
head and hair very well with
soap and with water in order to
wash away any pathogen that is
present in the hair and on the
skin. It is good to rub aloe vera
and olive oil on the hair and on
the skin. Aloe vera is very bitter,
this makes the skin and hair not

to be suitable for pathogens.

The olive oil makes the hair not

to break. When ever there is

symptom of head itch(pruritus),

it is good to wash the hair and

head with soap and clean water.

Itching of the head is early

symptom of disease occurrence.

25. Secrets about smoke: Smoke

is no healthy to the body.

Smoke contains free radicals.

What this free radicals does is

that they replace oxygen on the

hemoglobin in the blood.

Because of this the body will

not be well nourished. Smoking

of cigarette makes the lungs

and liver to change in color. This

is as a result of the black carbon

that is been taken in into the

body. This can result to

coughing. Smoke can mutate

the DNA of the lungs and liver.

This can cause cancer of the

liver and cancer of the lungs.

This makes the lungs and the

liver not to be healthy. The

lungs will not be able to

function properly in respiration

and the liver will not be able to

function properly in the storing

of blood, in detoxification and

in the digestion of food. The lips

and the sole of the feet will also

change in color when cigarette

is smoked. The lips will appear

dark and the feet will appear

dark. This is due to the black

carbon from the smoke of the

cigarette that is breathed into

the body.

26. Secrets about acid: Acid is

chemical that can burn without

flame. When it touches the skin

it burns it. This can cause the

skin to be burned away. It is

good to stay away from acid.

Apart of acid, very hot water

can cause the skin to burn. This

is because of the very high

temperature of heat from the

very hot water. When there is

very hot sun during the day,

when somebody stays under it

for very long time. It can cause

burn to the skin, which is sun

burn. This will lead to the

change of the color and

appearance. It can lead to skin

cancer and skin ulcer. It can

create room for disease causing

microorganisms to gain access

into the body. This is because

the injury that occur, disease

causing microorganisms can

invade it and infect it and also

further infect the inner parts of

the body. And the disease will

keep on spreading. It is

important to prevent this from

happening by going to the

hospital for therapy. Stay far

from acid, very hot water and

do not stay under the hot sun.

These helps to prevent skin

burn. The suitable temperature

for the body is 37 decree

Centigrade. When the

temperature then goes higher

than 37 degree centigrade it

cause fever. When the

temperature is very high it

cause skin burn. It is good to

have bath with water when the

body experience a little

temperature higher than

normal. Water is universal

coolant. It makes the body

temperature to come to normal.

But when there is burn on the

skin from the steam, it is good

to use egg and olive oil on it.

This can make the skin to easily

heal. It is good to take the

person immediately to the

hospital for therapy (treatment)

27. Secrets about sound: It is

good for sound to be normal.

This will make it not be too high

or too low for sound to be

heard normally. When the

sound is very high it cause

deafness. This is because of the

very high noise that is produced.

When the sound is very low, it is
difficult for the sound to be
heard or the sound will not be
heard. It is important to be far
from where there is very high
noise like quarry, that is where
they are breaking very big rocks.
When close to area where there
is breaking of very big rocks
without using aid that can
protect the ears. This can cause
deafness. It is good therefore

for those working in the place

where there is breaking of big

rocks to use ear aid that will

protect the ears from deafness.

It is also good for them to use

mask that will protect the nose.

This will help to filter dust away.

When dust is inhaled it cause

chest pain and cough. This is

because the dust enter into the

lungs. It is also good to use

spectacles that will protect dust

from entering the eyes, in order
to prevent eye infection and
disease. When there is dust in
the eyes, it can contains
pathogens that can cause
infection and disease to the
eyes. It can also cause itching
(pruritus) because the dust will
not make the eyes to be
comfortable. It is very good for
these to be prevented.